MEDICINAL HERBS FOR CANINE WELL-BEING

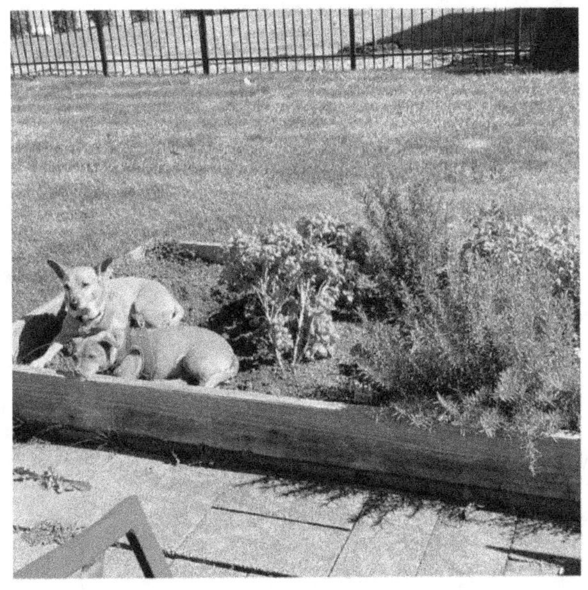

The Natural Way Encyclopedia and Guide to Improve Your Dog's Life.

EPIPHANY HUB PRINTS

TABLE OF CONTENT

Nausea

Fresh ginger or a powdered version can be an amazing remedy for solving the problems of vomiting and nausea in dogs. If your dog is easily car sick, give them a few drops of ginger root extract about 30 minutes before a car trip

INTRODUCTION

The book **"Medicinal Herbs for Canine Well-being"** shines as a source of natural healing and healthful care for man's best friend in a world where the pursuit of holistic well-being for our furry friends takes center stage. This ground-breaking manual is more than just a book; it's an immersive exploration of the world of therapeutic herbs that reveals the keys to improving the health and vitality of your dog.

Imagine living a life free from the limitations of common illnesses, where your beloved dog flourishes in optimum health. "Medicinal Herbs for Canine Well-Being" carries this promise as it leads you on an engrossing investigation of the powerful medicinal qualities present in nature's pharmacy. This extensive reference, which covers both traditional and contemporary herbal therapies, is proof of the ability of plants to provide your pet a healthy, balanced life.

This book, written with precision and care by well-known herbalists and specialists in canine wellbeing, is a labor of love. It expertly combines traditional knowledge with the most recent scientific findings to give you a road map for maximizing the remarkable therapeutic potential of herbs. As you turn the pages, you will learn about the medicinal properties of each herb as well as useful suggestions for incorporating them into your dog's regular regimen.

The process becomes a knowledge tapestry that helps you make wise decisions regarding the well-being of your dog. This guide is your reliable travel companion on the way to natural treatment, regardless of whether you want to address specific health issues or just improve your dog's general well-being.

More than just a book, "Medicinal Herbs for Canine Well-being" promises your four-legged dog a better, happier existence, one that starts with the transformative counsel found inside these pages and the knowledge of nature. Take advantage of the therapeutic properties of herbs and set out to maximize your dog's health.

CHAPTER ONE

Medicinal Herbs for Canine Well-being

With the help of our in-depth guide on medicinal herbs, find the organic route to your dog's health. We explore the realm of herbal therapies intended to improve the general health of your dog friend in this priceless resource. Medicinal herbs provide a comprehensive approach to pet care, dealing with everything from common health conditions to boosting vigor and lifespan.

Discover a range of herbs that have been carefully chosen for their therapeutic qualities, each of which supports a distinct area of your dog's health. Our guide gives you the knowledge you need to make wise decisions for your pet, from fostering tranquility and a glossy coat to assisting with digestion and joint health.

Discover how to grow therapeutic herbs in your house to provide a reliable and easily available source of natural treatments. We give you knowledge about the standards for choosing herbs and grow-care advice so you can actively participate in your dog's health path.

This article offers helpful guidance on incorporating medicinal herbs into your dog's everyday routine, going beyond simple information. Whether you are seeking preventive treatment or addressing specific health issues, our holistic approach guarantees your beloved pet a healthy balance.

With the help of the medicinal herbs included in this handbook, which is a reliable source for responsible pet owners looking for a kind and natural approach to canine health, you may harness the power of nature and improve your dog's well-being.

Benefits and Considerations for Canine Health

Holistic Healing: Discover the use of medicinal plants in a holistic manner to treat general health issues in dogs.

Natural Immune Support: Learn how some herbs can strengthen the immune system and make the body more resilient to disease.

Enrichment of Nutrients: Learn about the nutritional advantages of several herbs that give dogs vital vitamins and minerals.

Balanced Energy: Discover how using medicinal herbs can help keep pets in a state of balance and energy.

Considerations When Using Medicinal Herbs for Dogs

Dosage and Administration: Comprehensive information on the recommended dosages and modes of administration to guarantee efficacy without side effects.

Individual Sensitivities: Talk about issues pertaining to personal allergies and sensitivities, stressing the value of close observation when using herbal remedies.

Integration with Conventional Treatments: Advice on how to combine traditional veterinarian care with herbal therapies to promote a team-based, all-encompassing approach to canine health.

Consultation with Veterinarians: Stress the need of developing a collaborative and informed decision-making process by talking with veterinarians prior to introducing herbal remedies.

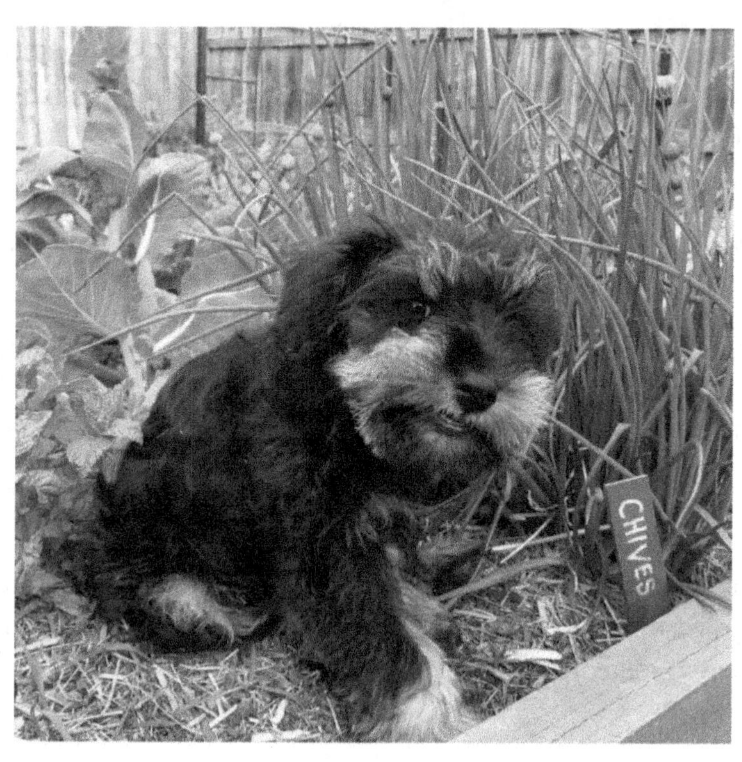

CHIVES

CHAPTER TWO
UNDERSTANDING CANINE HEALTH

Common Health Issues in Dogs

Overview of Common Health Issues: Learn about the most common health conditions that affect dogs, such as skin illnesses, allergies, digestive disorders, and joint issues.

Similar to people, dogs can have a variety of health problems that affect their general wellbeing. It's critical for pet owners to comprehend common health problems in order to identify symptoms early, seek veterinarian care promptly, and offer their furry friends the assistance they need.

We will discuss common health concerns that dogs have in this review, such as allergies, digestive issues, joint issues, and skin ailments.

Allergies:

Allergies can appear in a variety of ways and are a common health concern in dogs. Itching, redness, ear infections, and digestive problems can result from food allergies and environmental allergens including mold, dust mites, and pollen. Sneezing, licking, scratching, and upset stomach are typical symptoms.

Management:

Testing is used to identify allergies.

Dietary adjustments to get rid of possible food triggers.

Drugs that relieve symptoms, such as steroids or antihistamines.

Immune treatment for ongoing care.

Digestive Disorders

Infections, improper diet choices, and underlying medical conditions can all contribute to digestive problems in dogs. Constipation, diarrhea, vomiting, and inflammatory bowel disease are common digestive diseases. It's critical to keep a balanced diet and take quick action when experiencing gastrointestinal issues.

Management:

Diet modifications, like switching to a bland or hypoallergenic diet.

Probiotics to help maintain intestinal health.

pharmaceuticals to treat symptoms.

veterinarian consultation for a comprehensive diagnosis and course of care.

Joint Problems

Arthritis and hip dysplasia are two common joint issues, particularly in elderly dogs and some breeds. These ailments may result in pain, stiffness, and decreased range of motion. Age, trauma, and heredity can all contribute to joint issues.

Management:

Control your weight to ease joint strain.

Moderate activity on a regular basis to keep joints flexible.

supplements for joints that include chondroitin and glucosamine.

painkillers that a veterinarian has recommended.

Skin Conditions

Dog skin disorders can be brought on by fungi, parasites, allergies, or underlying medical conditions. Fungal infections, hot spots, and dermatitis are common skin conditions. Itching, redness, hair loss, and skin lesions are possible symptoms.

Management:

Regular hygiene and grooming regimens.

Therapy for underlying conditions (infections, allergies).

Topical treatments or medicated shampoos.

Nutritional supplements that support healthy skin.

Symptoms and Indicators:

Give advice on how to identify symptoms and indicators of common canine health problems so that early detection and treatment are possible.

Early detection increases the likelihood that a therapy will be successful and preserves the general health of the animal companions owned by pet owners. We will explore the main symptoms of common dog health problems in this book, enabling pet owners to be aware of and receptive to their dogs' medical requirements.

Digestive Issues

Symptoms: Includes constipation, diarrhea, vomiting often, changes in appetite, and lethargic behavior.

Indicators: Stool containing blood, abrupt weight loss, pain in the abdomen, and variations in water intake are all warning signs.

Common Problems: food intolerances, inflammatory bowel disease, and intestinal infections.

Joints and Mobility Issues

Symptoms: Include reduced activity levels, stiffness, trouble sitting or standing up, aversion to stairs and jumping, and limping.

Indicators: Pain during movement include visible indications such as swelling around joints and audible cracking or popping sounds.

Common Problems: Ligament injuries, hip dysplasia, and arthritis.

Dental Health Issues

Symptoms: Includes bad breath, swollen or bleeding gums, drooling excessively, and mouth pawing.

Indicators: Tartar accumulation, missing or loose teeth, and altered eating patterns are all warning signs.

Common Problems: Dental infections, gingivitis, and periodontal disease.

Coat and Skin Issues

Symptoms: Itching, redness, hair loss, dry or flaky skin, and textural changes in the coat are some of the symptoms.

Indicators: include rashes, the appearance of lumps or bumps, and unpleasant smells.

Common Issues: Allergies, rashes, and parasite infestations are common problems.

Respiratory Problems

Symptoms: Include nasal discharge, hard breathing, wheezing, sneezing, and coughing.

Indicators: Gums with a blue tint, a chronic cough, and an elevated respiratory rate are warning signs.

Common Problems: Allergies, heart issues, and respiratory infections.

Changes in Behavior

Symptoms: Anxiety, hostility, frequent barking, and irregular sleep patterns are some of the symptoms.

Indicators: Includes abrupt behavioral shifts, disengagement, and lack of interest in previous activities.

Common Problems: Cognitive decline, anxiety disorders, and behavioral abnormalities brought on by pain.

Kidney and Urinary Problems

Symptoms: Includes changes in water intake, fatigue, blood in the urine, and increased or decreased urination.

Indicators: Include straining to go to the bathroom, having mishaps at home, and experiencing pain when peeing.

Common Problems: Kidney illness, bladder stones, urinary tract infections.

Knowing the signs and symptoms of common dog health problems enables pet owners to take a proactive approach to their pets' wellbeing. Frequent veterinarian visits, careful monitoring of alterations in behavior, and quick attention to any indications of discomfort or suffering all help to provide the early identification and care required to preserve the best possible health for dogs.

Pet owners, via being watchful, responsive, and cultivating a close relationship with their vets, play a critical role in the health of their dogs.

Recognizing the Causes: Examine the underlying causes of common dog health disorders, stressing the significance of treating the core problems for long-term health.

Promoting long-term health and happiness in our beloved friends requires addressing the underlying causes rather than just treating the symptoms.

Numerous health problems can affect dogs, such as allergies, gastrointestinal disorders, skin disorders, obesity, and behavioral difficulties. Even while these concerns can take many different forms, they frequently have similar underlying causes that, if ignored, can result in chronic or recurrent health problems.

The Importance of Identifying Root Causes

While treating symptoms could offer short-term respite, doing so ignores the underlying causes of a dog's health concerns. A dog's general well-being cannot be sustained until the underlying problems are identified and addressed. This method is similar to treating an issue at its root as opposed to only addressing its external symptoms.

Allergies

Root Causes: Determining particular allergens or intolerances, such as substances, environments, or foods.

Importance: Adapting a dog's surroundings, food, and way of life to reduce or eliminate exposure to allergens is important.

Digestive Issues

Root Causes: Examining food quality, diet, and any possible gastrointestinal problems are the root causes.

Importance: Changing one's diet, taking care of dietary sensitivity issues, and encouraging a balanced gut flora are all crucial for better digestion.

Skin Issues

Root Causes; Examining underlying problems such as allergies, infections, or hormone abnormalities is known as root cause analysis.

Importance: Ensuring a pleasant and healthy coat by treating the underlying cause of skin problems.

Overweight

Root Causes: Examining one's food, level of exercise, and any possible underlying medical issues.

Importance: Implementing a healthy diet, engaging in regular exercise, and taking care of any underlying medical conditions that may be causing weight gain are all important.

Root Causes: Examining environmental influences, a deficiency of mental stimulation, or underlying medical issues are potential root causes.

Importance: Addressing any health conditions causing behavioral problems, offering mental enrichment, and providing proper training.

Implementing Solutions

Targeted solution implementation is more successful after the identification of the underlying reasons. This could entail nutritional modifications, way of life adjustments, behavior modification, and, if required, veterinary care. Ongoing monitoring and treatment plan modifications are ensured by routine examinations and honest conversation with veterinarians.

It is essential to comprehend the underlying reasons of prevalent health issues in dogs in order to support their long-term wellbeing. Together, pet owners and veterinarians may identify the underlying causes of symptoms and develop customized remedies that address the core problems, making canine companions happier, healthier, and more resilient. Proactively managing canine health guarantees our cherished companions a better standard of living.

Effect on Quality of Life

Talk about how typical health problems, such as discomfort or behavioral changes, might affect a dog's overall quality of life.

Common health problems can have a big impact on a dog's wellbeing, from behavioral abnormalities to physical discomfort. In this conversation, we examine how common health problems affect a dog's quality of life and stress the significance of prompt diagnosis, preventative measures, and all-encompassing treatment.

Physical Discomfort: **Problems with discomfort and Mobility:** Chronic discomfort and limited mobility in dogs can result from conditions like hip dysplasia, arthritis, or joint issues. This physical pain may make you less inclined to play, participate in activities, or even just move about comfortably.

Dental Problems: Untreated dental conditions like tooth decay or gum disease can make eating uncomfortable, which lowers energy and nutrition levels overall.

Digestive disorders: **Gastrointestinal Upset:** Dietary sensitivities, infections, or other gastrointestinal illnesses can cause dogs to have digestive problems such as vomiting, diarrhea, or constipation. These problems may include pain, fatigue, and a decline in appetite.

Skin Issues:

Itching and Irritation: Prolonged itching and skin irritation might be caused by allergies, dermatitis, or parasitic infestations. Constant discomfort can cause anxiety, restlessness, and behavioral problems.

Modifications in Behavior:

Aggression and Irritability: Aggression and irritability are two ways that chronic pain or discomfort can show up. In pain, a dog may respond defensively, which could impact how it interacts with people and other animals.

Depression and Lethargy: Lethargy and depression in dogs can be caused by long-term health problems. A dog that was previously lively and enthusiastic may show a discernible decrease in zeal and involvement.

Deficits in Sensations:

Loss of vision and hearing: Sensory deficits can be brought on by aging or specific medical diseases. Dogs that lose their hearing or eyesight may experience behavioral changes as they adjust to their new reality. They may also become confused or nervous.

Handling Chronic Illnesses: Dogs suffering from long-term ailments including diabetes, renal illness, or heart disease could need constant medical attention. A dog's general health might be impacted by the daily schedules related to medication, dietary restrictions, and veterinarian visits.

Responsible pet ownership requires an understanding of how common health problems affect a dog's quality of life. Preventive treatment, early intervention, and routine veterinary exams can help dogs stay healthier overall by lessening the consequences of health issues.

Through the management of both the physical and behavioral elements, pet owners may guarantee that their dogs live happy, healthy lives devoid of needless pain and suffering.

The Role of Medicinal Herbs in Addressing Common   Health Issues

1. Holistic Healing Approach:

Explain the idea of controlling and preventing common health concerns with medicinal herbs in a holistic manner.

Recognizing the interdependence of different facets of a dog's health, this holistic approach seeks to improve both the physical and mental state of health. In this talk, we examine the idea of treating common health problems in dogs holistically by managing and avoiding them with medicinal herbs.

Treatment of the full person is the goal of holistic medicine as opposed to addressing individual symptoms. It considers the elements that go into general well-being, such as environmental, emotional, and physical aspects. When it comes to dog care, this ideology calls for taking traditional medical treatments into account in addition to the dog's lifestyle, food, and emotional state.

Herbal Medicines with Healing Properties:

Anti-Inflammatory Properties: Its anti-inflammatory qualities Numerous therapeutic plants, like ginger and turmeric, have strong anti-inflammatory qualities. By lowering inflammation brought on by ailments like arthritis, these herbs can improve joint health and range of motion.

Adaptogenic Herbs: By assisting the body in adjusting to stimuli, adaptogenic herbs, such as holy basil and ashwagandha, foster resilience and equilibrium. These herbs may support dogs' emotional health and aid in the management of stress-related conditions.

Herbs that stimulate the Immune System: Echinacea and astragalus are well-known for their ability to stimulate the immune system. By adding these herbs to their diet, dogs' immune systems may be strengthened and given more defense against illnesses and infections.

Herbs and Digestive Health:

Herbs that Calm: Two herbs well-known for their relaxing properties are chamomile and lavender. For dogs that are having unsettled stomachs as a result of stress or anxiety, these herbs may be helpful.

Herbs for Digestive Aid: Fennel and peppermint are two herbs that can help with digestion and relieve symptoms like gas and bloating. Maintaining gut health enhances comfort and wellbeing in general.

Herbs for Healthy Skin and Coats:

Herbs having anti-allergenic qualities: Nettle and calendula are two examples of herbs that can help dogs with skin issues. These herbs might aid with itching relief and coat health.

Antimicrobial Herbs: By treating bacterial or fungal diseases, antimicrobial herbs like thyme and oregano help improve the health of your skin.

Pharmaceutical Herbs for Preventive Care:

Herbal Supplementation: Including therapeutic herbs in a dog's food on a regular basis can help guard against common health problems. This proactive strategy fosters long-term wellbeing and strengthens the body's natural defenses.

The tenets of holistic care are supported by the use of medicinal herbs as a holistic treatment strategy for treating and preventing common health problems in dogs. Natural remedies can be used in addition to traditional veterinary treatments by pet owners who take into account the physical, emotional, and preventive elements of canine health.

Nonetheless, it's essential to confer with herbalists as well as veterinarians to guarantee a secure, well-rounded strategy catered to each dog's unique requirements. Including medicinal herbs in a comprehensive care plan shows that we are dedicated to our dogs' general health and vigor.

2   Particular   Herb-Health Connections:

Make links between particular herbs and how well they work to treat particular common health issues. Examples include herbs for skin diseases, allergies, and joint support.

In this research, we focus on particular herb-health relationships, demonstrating how well-suited some herbs are to common canine health issues like allergies, joint support, and skin ailments.

Allergies:

Matricaria chamomilla, or chamomile: Chamomile is well known for its sedative and anti-inflammatory qualities. Chamomile can help dogs with allergies feel less itchy and irritated on their skin. Applying chamomile topically or taking it as a supplement helps reduce allergic symptoms.

Nettle (Urtica dioica): Nettle is good for dogs who have symptoms related to allergies because it has antihistamine qualities. It can ease typical allergic reactions by reducing inflammation and itching.

Joint Support:

Turmeric (Curcuma longa): Curcumin, the key ingredient in turmeric (Curcuma longa), has strong anti-inflammatory properties. When it comes to arthritis-related joint pain and stiffness, turmeric can help. For elderly or arthritic dogs, it enhances joint health and increases mobility.

Boswellia (Boswellia serrata): Boswellia is known to have anti-inflammatory properties that support healthy joints. Its ability to lower inflammation and improve overall joint function makes it very helpful in the management of disorders such as osteoarthritis.

Skin Issues:

Calendula (Calendula officinalis): Calendula is helpful in treating a variety of skin diseases since it has anti-inflammatory and antibacterial qualities. It can be administered topically to relieve discomfort, encourage healing, and calm irritated skin.

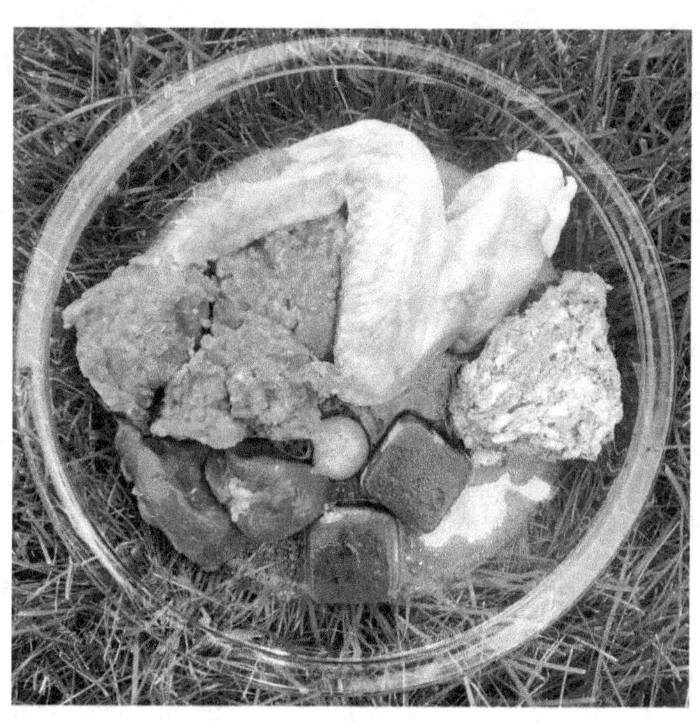

Burdock Root (Arctium lappa): Burdock root has a reputation for being a detoxifier and is useful in treating skin disorders brought on by pollutants or toxins. By addressing the underlying causes of skin problems, it promotes healthy skin and coat.

Digestive disorders

The digestive advantages of peppermint (Mentha × piperita) are well-known. Peppermint leaves dogs with digestive problems feeling less bloated and with dyspepsia. It soothes the gastrointestinal system.

Ginger (Zingiber officinale): Ginger helps with digestion and is good for dogs that have upset stomachs or nausea. It may lessen the symptoms of a number of digestive diseases and aid in calming the digestive tract.

Pet owners can use medicinal herbs to treat common health issues in their dogs by knowing the unique relationships between herbs and health. Under the supervision of veterinarians and herbalists, adding these herbs to a dog's regimen of care can offer safe, all-natural treatments.

To guarantee the safety and suitability of herbal medicines for certain canines, it is imperative to consult veterinary professionals as with any health-related action.

3 Preventive Measures:

To reduce the likelihood of frequent health issues, emphasize the preventive advantages of adding medicinal herbs to a dog's daily routine.

Medicinal herbs can be incorporated into a dog's regimen as a preventative measure against common health issues. In this talk, we explore the preventive advantages of medicinal herbs and highlight their function in treating and preventing possible health problems in our dog friends.

Support for the Immune System:

Herbs such as Echinacea and Astragalus: Herbs that are known to strengthen the immune system include astragalus and echinacea. Frequent supplementing helps strengthen the dog's defenses against disease and infection.

Anti-Inflammatory Effects:

Boswellia and Turmeric: Are examples of medicinal plants with anti-inflammatory qualities that can help reduce inflammation, which is frequently linked to illnesses like arthritis. These herbs support joint health by lowering inflammation, which may also delay the onset of chronic pain.

Digestive Tract health

Peppermint and Ginger: Herbs with digestive properties, like peppermint and ginger, can help keep the gastrointestinal tract in good condition. By preventing problems like bloating, diarrhea, and indigestion, they may help guarantee the best possible absorption of nutrients.

Dental Health:

Neem and Parsley: Certain herbs, like parsley and neem, naturally possess antibacterial qualities that promote oral health. By include these herbs in a dog's routine, you can lower the risk of discomfort and possible systemic health problems associated with periodontal disorders.

Protection from Antioxidants:

Herbs high in antioxidants, such as oregano and rosemary, can fight free radicals, which are linked to aging and a number of health issues. Frequent consumption of these herbs can protect cells and improve the health of the dog as a whole.

Reducing Stress:

Chamomile and Lavender: Herbs with relaxing properties like chamomile and lavender can help dogs cope with stress and anxiety. Reducing stress has advantages for behavioral health as well as the potential to prevent health problems associated with stress.

Preventing Parasites:

Garlic and Thyme: Some plants have inherent qualities that could discourage parasites. Using these herbs can be an extra line of defense against parasites, even if veterinary advice is still essential for parasite prevention.

Dong Quai with Red Clover: The health of the reproductive system depends on hormonal balance. Herbs used medicinally that have adaptogenic qualities may help maintain hormonal balance and lower the chance of reproductive problems.

4 Complementary Strategies:

Talk about how using herbal medicines in addition to traditional veterinary care can help dogs stay healthy overall.

Although traditional veterinarian care is essential for identifying and treating certain conditions, herbal remedies provide something special for general health.

Supportive Wellness: Taking herbal medications can help avoid a number of health problems by strengthening the immune system, promoting vitality, and enhancing overall health.

These homeopathic treatments, when combined with routine veterinary examinations, offer a holistic approach to wellness that addresses current issues while building resistance to future hardships.

Minimizing Side Effects: Conventional drugs occasionally have side effects. Using herbal supplements sparingly can help lessen these symptoms and provide a more harmonious and well-balanced treatment approach. Dogs can receive treatments with more comfort and less stress by reducing the impact of adverse reactions.

Addressing Root Causes: Rather than only treating symptoms, herbal treatments frequently address the underlying causes of health problems. This proactive approach, which aims to address bodily imbalances before they become clinical issues, is consistent with the concepts of preventative care.

Including herbal remedies in the regimen promotes a more thorough comprehension and control of your dog's health.

Maintaining Holistic Health: A holistic approach to health is beneficial for both humans and dogs. Herbal remedies help with this by boosting mental and emotional health in addition to treating physical problems. Herbal supplements offer a range of holistic advantages that go beyond the physical, such as enhancing cognitive function or relieving anxiety.

Customized Solutions: Since every dog is different, herbal remedies provide a wide range of solutions that can be adjusted to meet specific requirements. With this tailored approach, you can be confident that your dog will receive a treatment plan that meets their unique health needs, leading to a more efficient and individualized care routine.

A dynamic collaboration that optimizes the potential for canine well-being is created when herbal medicines are combined with conventional veterinarian care. This complementary approach combines the best aspects of both fields, utilizing the accuracy of veterinary medicine and the holistic knowledge of herbal treatments to help your beloved pet live a healthy, happy, and robust life.

The purpose of this chapter is to improve the reader's comprehension of frequent canine health problems and the function that medicinal herbs play in fostering and preserving general canine health.

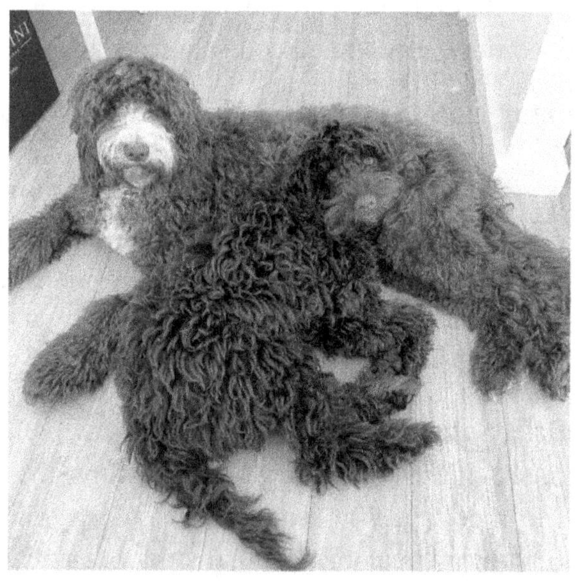

CHAPTER THREE

SELECTING AND GROWING MEDICINAL HERBS

Criteria for Choosing Herbs

Choosing and cultivating medicinal herbs for dogs involves giving careful thought to a number of factors in order to protect the health of the pets. The following are some crucial things to remember:

Dog Safety:

Verify that the herbs you've chosen are safe for your dog to eat. Certain herbs that are good for people could be poisonous to dogs. Prior to adding any herbs to your dog's diet, be sure they are safe by double-checking the information with reliable sources.

Health Benefits:

Select herbs that are particularly beneficial to dogs' health. Herbs that can help with skin disorders include calendula and chamomile, which have anti-inflammatory qualities, and ginger, which can help with digestion.

Compatibility with Canine Diet:

Select herbs that meet your dog's nutritional demands while keeping in mind their dietary needs. While certain herbs work better in therapeutic teas or tinctures, others can be put to dog food or treats.

Ease of Growth:

Choose herbs that are locally easy to grow. Herbs that grow well in your region's soil and climate will need less care and offer a steady supply of therapeutic plants.

Non-Invasive Growth:

Choose herbs that won't harm the surrounding vegetation or other plants in your garden. Certain herbs have the potential to become invasive, taking over the garden and endangering other plant species.

Steer clear of harmful pesticides:

When cultivating plants for therapeutic uses, it's crucial to stay away from dangerous pesticides. Use organic growing techniques to guarantee that the herbs don't contain any possibly harmful materials.

Speaking with a veterinarian:

See a veterinarian prior to adding any therapeutic herbs to a dog's diet. A specialist can offer advice regarding your dog's unique medical requirements and whether or not certain herbs are suitable for them.

Warnings and Restrictions:

Recognize any warnings or restrictions related to particular plants. It's important to be aware of the potential hazards associated with some herbs as they may interact with drugs or make certain health conditions worse.

Procedures for Harvesting:

In order to preserve the sustainability of the herbs, gather them responsibly. To optimize the medicinal benefits of herbs, harvest them at the ideal time. Avoid overharvesting to enable the plants to regenerate.

Storage and Drying:

To keep the gathered herbs potent, store and dry them properly. This guarantees that you will always have an ample supply of healing herbs for your dog.

By taking these factors into account, you may establish a secure and advantageous environment for cultivating and using medicinal herbs for your dogs' health. When adding herbs to your pet's care routine, always put their health and wellbeing first.

Tips for Cultivating Medicinal Herbs at Home

Growing therapeutic herbs at home for your dog's health can be a fulfilling and advantageous effort. The following advice will help you choose and cultivate medicinal herbs that are specifically beneficial to your dog's health:

Examine Herbs Safe for Dogs:

Do your homework on dog-safe plants before you grow them. Certain herbs may even be toxic to dogs, therefore not all of them are good to eat. Emphasize on herbs that are safe for dogs and have been shown to have medical benefits.

Speak with Your Vet:

Before adding any new herbs to your dog's diet, make sure to speak with your veterinarian. They can offer advice on particular herbs that can help your dog's health issues and make sure the herbs you choose won't have any unfavorable interactions with any pharmaceuticals you currently take.

Establish a Dog-Friendly Garden Area:

Set aside a certain section of your garden to grow herbs for your dog. Ensure that it is both conveniently located for your pet and sufficiently safe to keep them from inadvertently eating potentially dangerous plants.

Choose Easy-to-cultivate Herbs:

Pick herbs that are simple to cultivate and care for. Herbs like parsley, calendula, and chamomile may be included in this. Make sure the soil, water, and sunshine levels are appropriate for the particular requirements of each herb.

Use Organic Fertilizers and Soil:

To keep your dog safe from dangerous chemicals, choose organic fertilizers and soil. This guarantees that the herbs cultivated are as healthy and natural as possible.

Harvest and Inspect Frequently:

Check your herb garden frequently for indications of illness or pest activity. Deal with problems as soon as possible to keep the supply of herbs healthy. To optimize the medicinal benefits of herbs, gather them at their prime.

Dry and Store Herbs Correctly:

To maintain the therapeutic properties of collected herbs, dry and store them correctly. Pick a technique that works for each herb, such as dehydrating or air drying. The dried herbs should be kept in a dark, cool place.

Add Herbs to Dog's food:

Gradually add therapeutic herbs to your dog's food after you have a sufficient supply on hand. Start with little quantities and see how your dog reacts. Herbs can be used to prepare herbal teas or added to food.

Examine Your Dog's Behavior:

Keep a tight eye on your dog's reaction to the herbs. Consult your veterinarian and stop using the product if you observe any negative responses. It's important to keep an eye on your dog's health because certain dogs may be sensitive to certain herbs.

Alternate Herbs Depending on Your Needs:

Choose your herbs according to the particular health requirements of your dog. For instance, concentrate on herbs recognized for their digestive advantages if your dog has digestive problems. Rotate your herb collection to offer a range of therapeutic benefits.

These pointers will help you design a dog-friendly herb garden that naturally and holistically improves the health of your furry pet. Always put your dog's health first, and seek the opinion of a veterinarian for specific recommendations.

CHAPTER FOUR

HERBS FOR DIGESTIVE HEALTH

Chamomile to relax the Stomach

Chamomile is widely known for its ability to relax, and this effect also extends to the digestive system. The active ingredients in chamomile, like bisabolol and chamazulene, have anti-spasmodic and anti-inflammatory qualities.

Because of these properties, chamomile is a great option for calming an upset stomach and easing discomfort related to digestion. One common way to ingest this herb is via chamomile tea, which is pleasant on the stomach due to its mild flavor.

Peppermint for Indigestion

It is commonly known that peppermint can relieve indigestion and support healthy digestion. The menthol in peppermint leaves the gastrointestinal tract feeling more relaxed, which lessens symptoms like gas, bloating, and indigestion.

It's normal to consume peppermint oil or peppermint tea. However, it's important to utilize peppermint carefully because some people may have heartburn if they consume too much of it.

Dandelion for Liver Support:

Dandelion is a powerful herb with several health benefits, one of which being liver support. It's not just your average weed. It has long been known that the root of the dandelion plant can stimulate the liver and encourage bile flow. Detoxification and digestion may benefit from this.

Dandelion leaves are a nutrient-dense addition to salads since they are high in vitamins and minerals. Drinking dandelion tea or including dandelion in your diet can benefit your liver in general.

Herbal Remedies for Dogs' Digestive Health:

Dogs' general health depends on maintaining their digestive systems. The digestive system of dogs may benefit from the use of certain therapeutic herbs:

Peppermint (Safe for Dogs): Peppermint has benefits for digestive problems in dogs that are comparable to those it has for people. Introduce tiny amounts by giving them snacks or by sprinkling a little bit of fresh mint leaves on their meals.

Ginger (Safe for Dogs): Ginger has anti-inflammatory qualities that can help dogs feel less queasy and calm their digestive systems. You can give it to them as treats or grated and added to their meals.

Parsley (Safe for Dogs): Parsley can help dogs digest food better and have less flatulence. It's okay to add this herb to their food or give them as a special treat from time to time.

Marshmallow Root (Ask a Vet): Marshmallow root has the potential to relieve gastrointestinal tract discomfort. It is important, nevertheless, to speak with a veterinarian before adding it to your dog's diet.

Prior to adding new herbs to your dog's food, always get advice from a veterinarian because different pets have different sensitivities and medical concerns. Furthermore, moderation is essential to guarantee the herbs' positive effects are balanced by their negative ones.

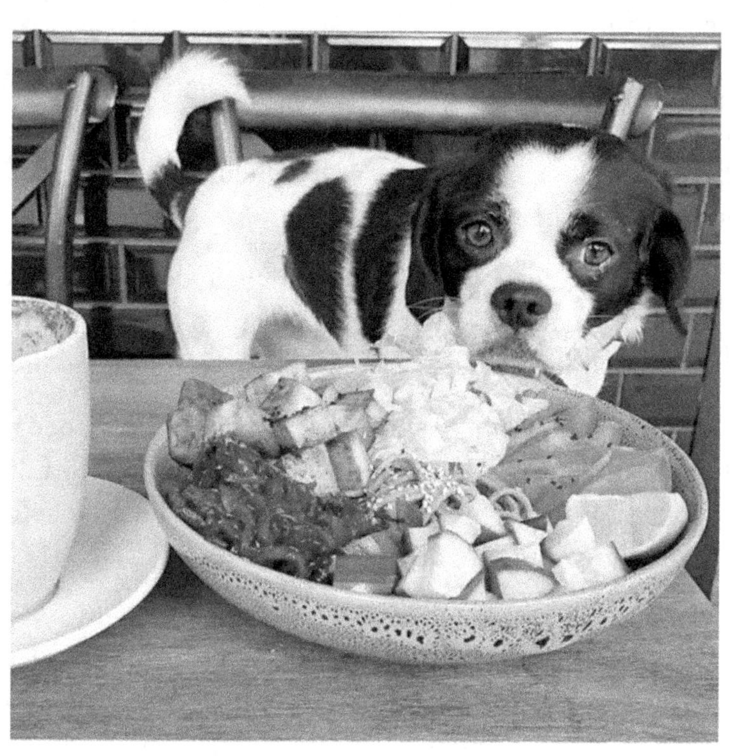

CHAPTER FIVE

HERBS FOR JOINT AND MOBILITY SUPPORT

Turmeric for Anti-inflammatory Benefits:

The bright yellow spice turmeric has become well-known for its strong anti-inflammatory qualities. Curcumin, the main ingredient in turmeric, is well known for its capacity to stop several inflammatory processes, therefore reducing inflammation. Research indicates that turmeric might be useful in treating inflammatory diseases like arthritis and other inflammatory ailments. Adding turmeric to your food or taking supplements could provide anti-inflammatory benefits without harming your body.

Devil's Claw for the Relief of Joint Pain:

The plant commonly referred to as Devil's Claw, or Harpagophytum procumbens, is indigenous to Southern

Africa. Devil's claw has long been utilized in herbal therapy and is now known to have the ability to reduce joint pain and stiffness. Compounds in the plant with anti-inflammatory qualities may aid in the treatment of rheumatoid arthritis and osteoarthritis. Devil's claw is a natural remedy for joint pain since it comes in a variety of forms, such as capsules and topical treatments.

Alfalfa for Supplemental Nutrients:

A nutrient-dense herb known for its abundance of vitamins and minerals is alfalfa. This herb is rich in several B vitamins and other nutrients such vitamins A, C, E, and K. Alfalfa is also an excellent provider of nutrients, including iron, magnesium, and calcium.

Adding alfalfa to your diet or taking supplements can help support your body's overall nutritional needs. But before adding alfalfa to your regimen, it's crucial to speak with a healthcare provider, particularly if you have any underlying medical concerns.

Herbs for Canines to Help with Joints and Mobility:

For our canine friends, several herbs may also help with joints and movement. Dogs' joint pain can be reduced by using herbs with anti-inflammatory qualities, such as boswellia, yucca, and meadowsweet.

These herbs can be given to dogs as part of their diet or added to supplements made especially for them, after consulting a veterinarian. It is imperative to confirm that any herbal supplements prescribed for dogs are suitable and safe for their individual medical requirements.

See a doctor or veterinarian before adding any herbs or supplements to your regimen, particularly if you have any underlying medical ailments or are concerned about the health of your pet. Furthermore, each person will react to herbs differently, so it's important to be aware of any possible drug or allergy combinations.

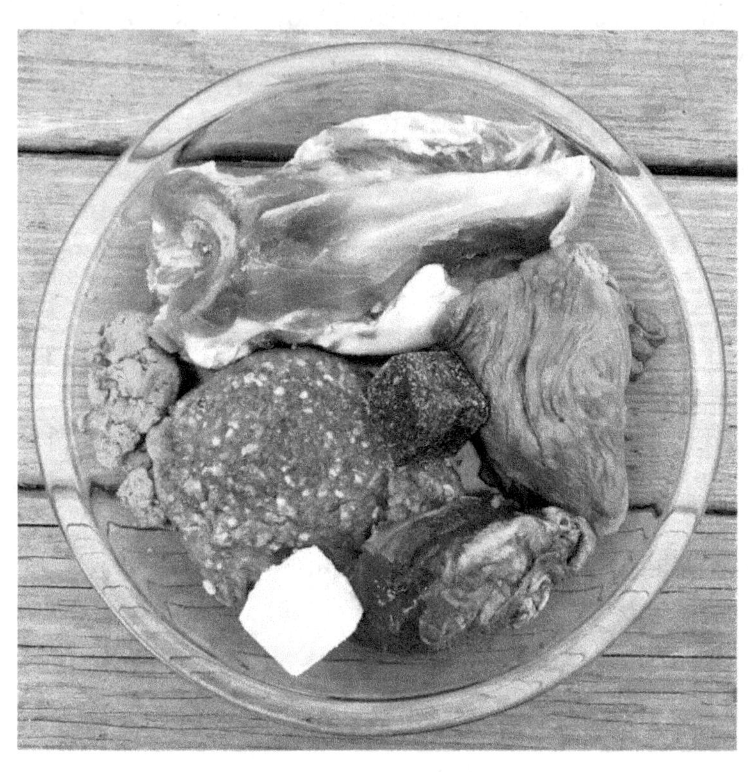

CHAPTER SIX

HERBS FOR SKIN AND COAT HEALTH

Aloe Vera for Skin Irritations:

Aloe Vera is a well-known natural medicine that is great for relieving skin irritations because of its calming qualities. Its gel, which is extracted from the succulent Aloe Vera leaves, has cooling and anti-inflammatory properties. Aloe Vera can help with a variety of skin issues, including sunburn, rashes, and small burns, when applied topically.

By hydrating and moisturizing the skin, the gel hastens healing and lessens irritation. Aloe Vera also possesses antibacterial qualities that might help shield against infections brought on by skin irritations. Apply the gel directly to the irritated region of skin and let it absorb to utilize aloe vera for skin irritations.

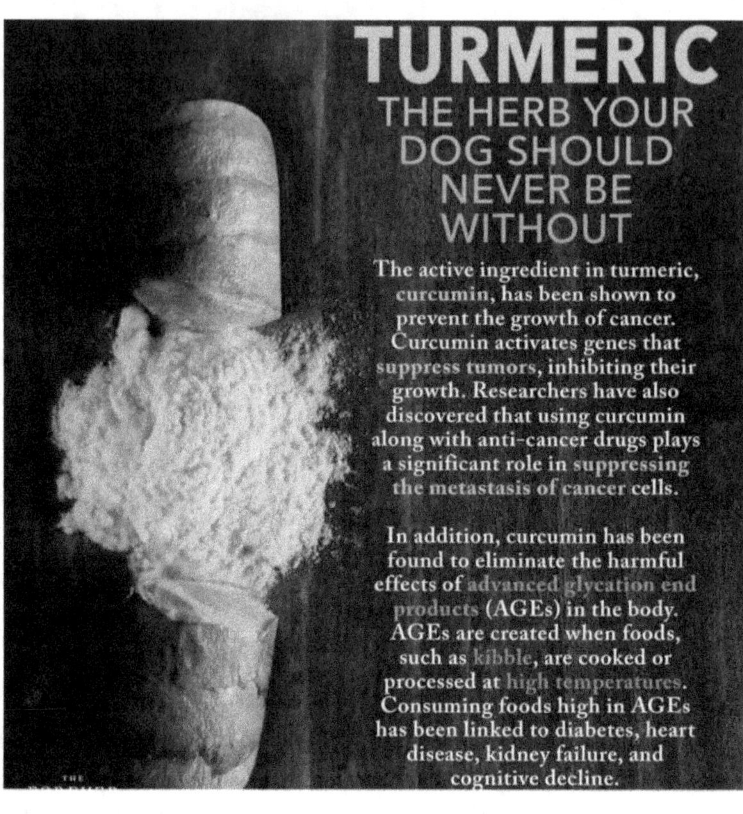

Burdock Root to Condition Coats:

The burdock plant yields burdock root, a herbal medicine that is beneficial for conditioning pet coats in many ways. Burdock Root, which is high in vital fatty acids, helps nourish the skin and coat and encourages a radiant, healthy appearance. It is especially helpful for dogs whose skin is flaky or dry since it helps them stay hydrated and lessens itching.

The root contains substances that improve overall coat texture and prevent dryness, giving the coat a lustrous, smooth finish. Burdock Root can be added to your pet's diet in a number of ways, including teas, capsules, and specialty pet meals. Utilizing burdock root on a regular basis can help you keep your dog's coat healthy and colorful.

Calendula's Healing Properties for the Health of Canine Skin and Coats:

Calendula, often known as marigold, is a plant with amazing healing qualities. It is a great option to support the health of your dog's skin and coat. Anti-inflammatory and antibacterial substances found in calendula extracts help calm irritated skin, lessen redness, and promote healing.

Dogs with small wounds, abrasions, or skin irritations may benefit from the application of calendula in topical ointments, shampoos, or as an infused oil. Regular usage can help maintain a robust and healthy coat, and its soft nature makes it suited for delicate skin. Calendula is a natural solution for pet owners who want to improve their dogs' general health and manage skin problems.

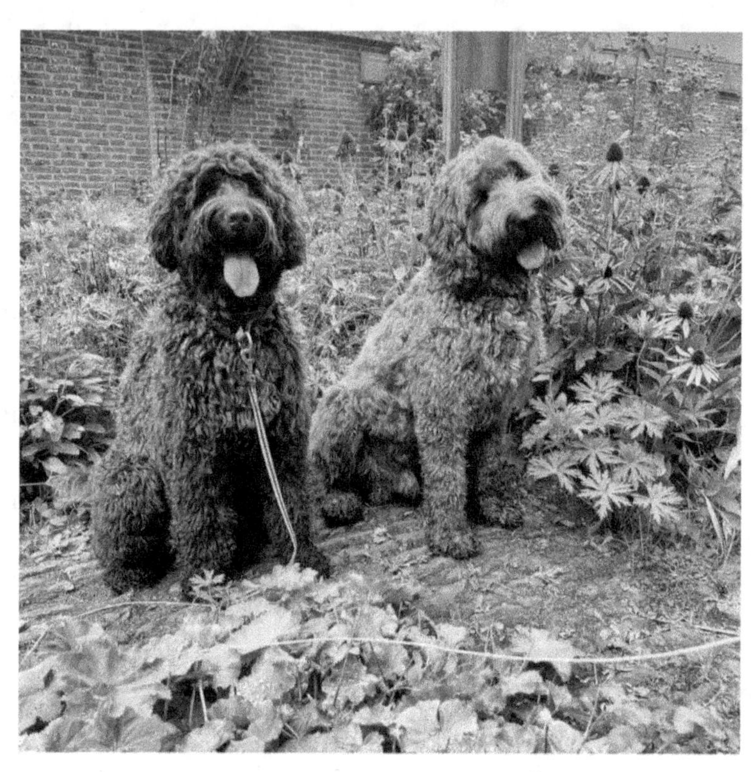

CHAPTER SEVEN

HERBS FOR RESPIRATORY HEALTH

Eucalyptus for Respiratory Support:

Eucalyptus is widely utilized to maintain respiratory health in both humans and dogs because of its well-known respiratory advantages. Compounds like cineole, which are found in eucalyptus leaves, are present in the essential oil that is extracted from them and can facilitate easier breathing.

Application: To create an environment that is conducive to dogs' respiratory systems, eucalyptus oil can be diluted, diffused, or added to a humidifier. To prevent any negative effects, it is imperative to guarantee adequate dilution.

Using Licorice Root to Treat Sore Throat:

Licorice root is frequently used to relieve sore throats due to its inherent anti-inflammatory qualities. For dogs who are coughing or have irritation in their throats, it may be helpful.

Application: You can add licorice root to your dog's food or water, or steep it into a tea (after it cools). It's important to take licorice root in moderation because taking too much of it can have unfavorable side effects.

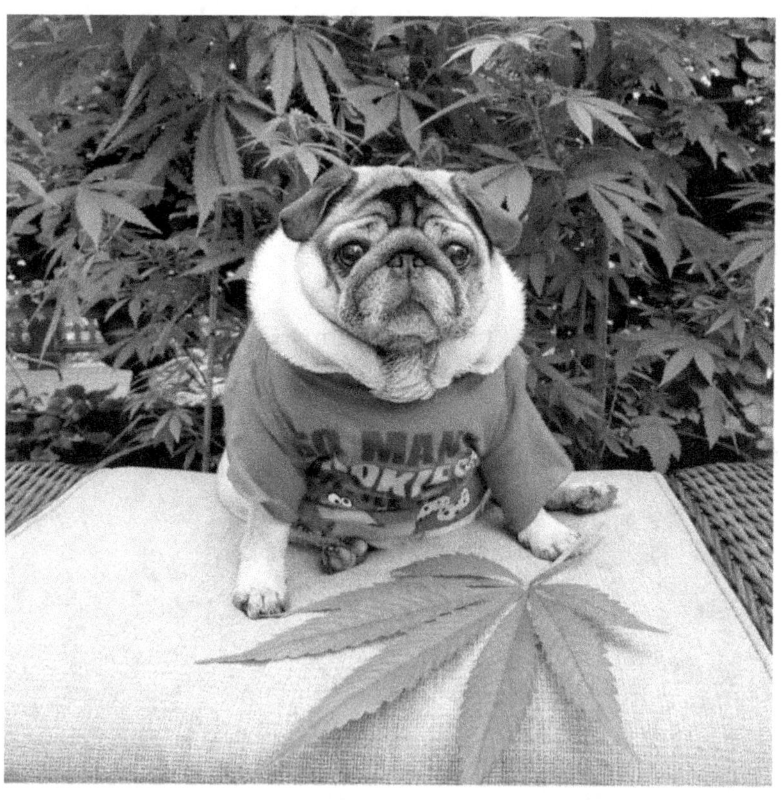

Mullein in Support of Respiratory Health:

Mullein is a plant with a reputation for helping respiratory issues. It is thought to offer calming qualities that can support a dog's respiratory health. Mullein is frequently used to treat conditions including congestion and coughing.

Application: Mullein can be brewed as a tea and put in your dog's food or water. As an alternative, there can be commercial mullein supplements made especially for canines.

Note: It's important to see a veterinarian before adding any herbal therapies to your dog's regimen. Some dogs may have pre-existing problems or sensitivities that could be affected, and not all dogs may respond to these therapies in the same manner.

To protect your pet's safety and wellbeing, you should also talk to a veterinarian about the right dosage and method of administration.

Bloating:

Ginger helps in relieving or preventing bloat in dogs due to its ability to stimulate movement in the stomach and accelerate emptying of the stomach (demonstrated in several studies).

CHAPTER EIGHT
HERBS FOR ANXIETY AND STRESS

Commonly used herbs that are well-known for their calming, relaxing, and nerve-relieving qualities are lavender, passionflower, and Valerian. These herbs have the potential to help dogs feel more at ease and content when it comes to anxiety and stress. Here is a quick synopsis of each:

The Calming Effects of Valerian:

Description: Valerian has long been used for its relaxing and soothing properties.

Benefits for Dogs: It can ease a dog's anxiousness and anxiety while fostering calmness.

Application: Valerian root is frequently found in herbal supplements and as a component of dog treats that are meant to soothe anxiety.

Lavender Oil for Calm Mind:

Description: Known for its calming and relaxing effects, lavender is a fragrant herb.

Benefits for Dogs: Lavender helps reduce stress and encourage relaxation in dogs by helping to create a peaceful environment.

Application: Diluted lavender essential oil can be applied topically to a dog's bedding or collar. There are other dog products with lavender added.

Passionflower Reduction for Anxiety:

Description: The herb known as passionflower has a relaxing effect and is frequently used to ease anxiety and stress.

Benefits for Dogs: Passionflower supports a more composed temperament by calming anxiety and restlessness in dogs.

Application: Herbal remedies designed to alleviate anxiety in dogs frequently contain passionflower.

While some herbs may be helpful, it's important to remember that you should always see a veterinarian before starting any new supplement or treatment. The particular requirements and health state of each dog should be taken into consideration when determining the right dosage and mode of administration.

These herbs should also be utilized in conjunction with a healthy diet, regular exercise, and a stress-free environment as part of an all-encompassing strategy for canine wellbeing.

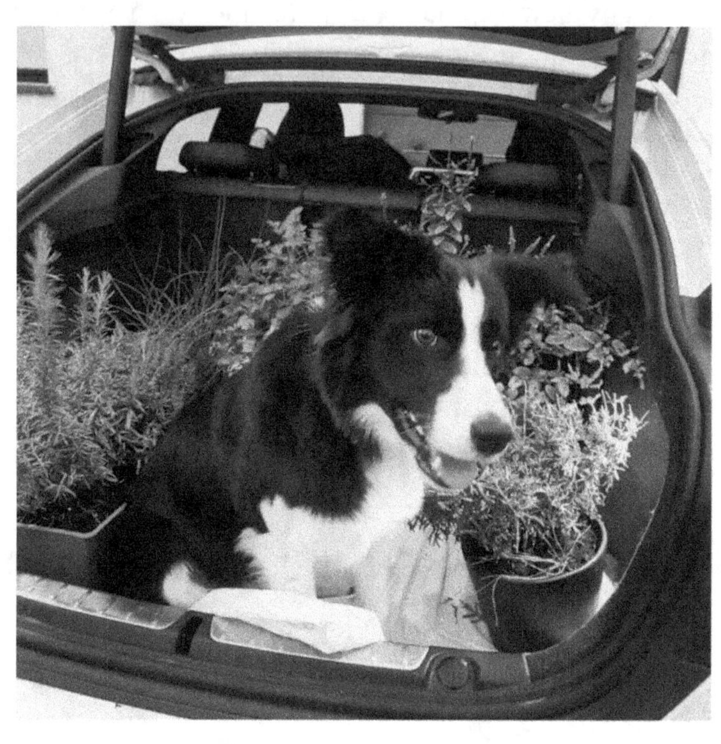

CHAPTER NINE
SAFETY CONSIDERATIONS AND DOSAGES

For millennia, people have utilized medicinal herbs to enhance their overall health and wellness. Although there may be advantages to using these natural cures, care must be taken when using them.

With an emphasis on possible interactions, side effects, and dosage recommendations to guarantee the highest level of safety and effectiveness, this guide offers crucial instructions for the responsible use of medicinal plants.

Consultation with Qualified Healthcare Professionals:

See a qualified healthcare practitioner before introducing any medicinal herbs into your regimen. Based on your unique health situation, current medications, and any potential contraindications, they can offer tailored advise.

Possible Interactions:

a. Drug Interactions: Recognize that there may be a conflict between prescription or over-the-counter drugs and medicinal herbs. Certain medications may have unfavorable interactions if certain herbs increase or decrease their effects.

b. Herb-Herb Interactions: The efficacy or unintended side effects of specific herbal combinations may be impacted by their interactions with one another. Before combining different herbs, look into possible interactions.

Side Effects:

a. Allergic responses: Keep an eye out for any allergic responses, including swelling, itching, or rashes on the skin. If you experience any allergy symptoms, stop using it right once.

b. Effects on the Gastrointestinal System: Certain herbs may result in gastrointestinal problems such nausea, vomiting, or diarrhea. Observe your body's reaction and modify the dosage as necessary.

c. Effects on the Central Nervous System: Some herbs have the potential to affect the central nervous system, which could result in mood swings, drowsiness, or dizziness. Be cautious, especially when driving or operating machinery.

Dosage Guidelines:

a. Start Low: If required, start with a low dosage and progressively raise it. This lessens the possibility of negative reactions and enables your body to adapt to the effects of the herb.

a. Comply with Suggested Guidelines: Make sure you follow any dose recommendations made by medical professionals or other reliable sources. Don't self-prescribe; instead, get advice on how much is right for your particular needs.

c. Track Individual Response: Observe how the herbal medicine affects your body's reaction. Individual reactions can differ, so it's critical to modify dosage in accordance with tolerance.

Quality and Source:

a. Select High-Quality Products: To guarantee quality and purity, use medicinal herbs from reliable suppliers. Low-quality items may contain adulterants or contaminants that exacerbate negative effects.

c. Fresh vs. Dried: Evaluate if the herb is better suited for your purposes in its fresh or dried state. The potency of fresh herbs may differ from that of their dried equivalents.

When done carefully and thoughtfully, using medicinal herbs can be a useful component of a holistic treatment strategy. Through consideration of possible interactions, careful monitoring for adverse effects, and adherence to recommended dosage guidelines, people can improve the security and efficacy of utilizing medicinal herbs for their overall health and well-being. For individualized guidance catered to your particular health profile, always seek the assistance of healthcare professionals.

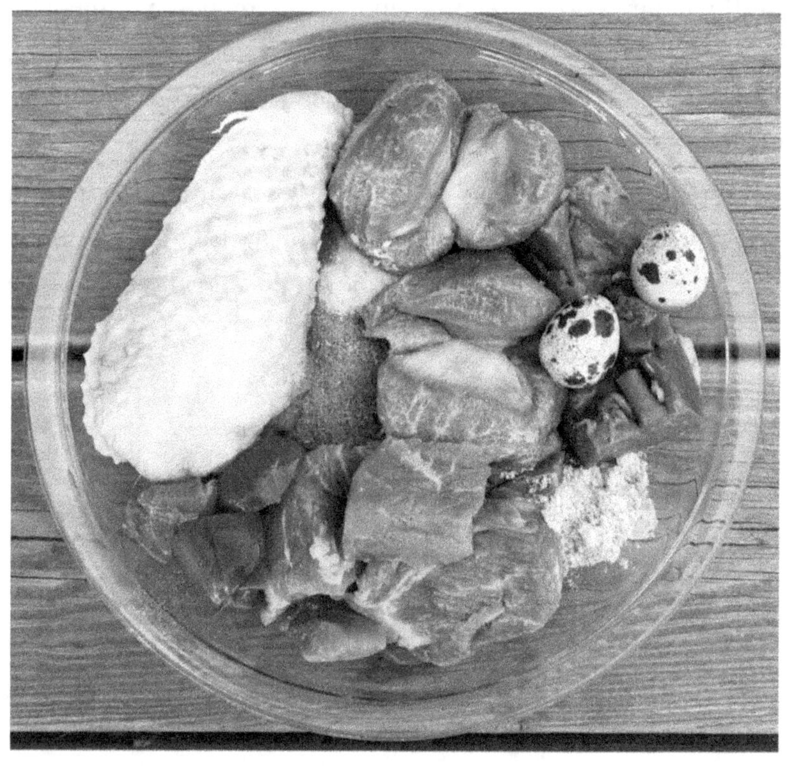

CHAPTER TEN

HOLISTIC APPROACH TO CANINE WELL-BEING

The use of medicinal herbs in the overall care of dogs has grown in popularity as pet owners look more and more for natural and holistic solutions to their dogs' health. Working together with both conventional doctors and skilled herbalists, this holistic approach guarantees a thorough and well-rounded approach to your dog's health.

The Function of Medicinal Herbs in the Health of Dogs:

For millennia, people have utilized medicinal plants to treat a range of health issues, and our dog friends can also benefit from these uses. Herbs with anti-inflammatory, immune-stimulating, and antioxidant qualities include chamomile, echinacea, and turmeric. Including these herbs in your dog's routine care can improve their general health and well-being.

Collaboration with Veterinarians:

It's important to speak with a licensed veterinarian before giving your dog therapeutic herbs. Veterinarians are qualified to assess your dog's unique medical requirements and make sure that any herbal supplements you give him are suitable and safe. They can also provide advice on how much to take and any possible drug interactions.

Important things to think about before seeing a veterinarian:

Provide a thorough history of your dog's medical conditions.

Talk about any current health problems or worries.

Tell others about your dog's diet and way of life.

Ask for advice on herbal supplements that suit the specific requirements of your dog.

Working Together with Herbalists:

Herbalists can provide significant insights into creating herbal medicines that are specifically matched to your dog's needs and bring expert knowledge of medicinal plants to the table. Traditional and tried-and-true herbal treatments can be included into the holistic approach to canine care when working with a competent herbalist.

Important things to think about before seeing a herbalist:

Select a respectable, knowledgeable herbalist who specializes in animal health.

Talk about the unique health objectives and worries for your dog.

Work together to develop a personalized herbal care regimen.

For a coordinated strategy, make sure the veterinarian and herbalist are in constant communication.

Integration and Monitoring:

It's critical to incorporate the advice of both a veterinarian and a herbalist into your dog's regular regimen after consulting with them both. Maintaining a close eye on your dog's health and any behavioral changes will assist determine how well the herbal therapies are working and enable any necessary adjustments.

Working with veterinarians and herbalists to incorporate medicinal herbs into general canine care provides a comprehensive and well-rounded approach to promoting your dog's health.

You can give your dog friend comprehensive and individualized treatment by fusing the knowledge of herbal remedies with the skill of traditional veterinary medicine. Always put your dog's health first by consulting a specialist and keeping lines of communication open between all parties.

CONCLUSION

Investigating natural and holistic alternatives to our beloved dogs' health becomes essential in a society where their welfare is our top priority. Embark on a captivating journey with us through "Medicinal Herbs for Canine Well-Being," a meticulously crafted handbook that empowers dog owners with the knowledge and techniques to harness the incredible healing power of nature.

We work hard to give our four-legged pals the finest care possible as their guardians, and this book is your reliable ally in this endeavor. This guide, which explores the amazing world of medicinal plants, goes beyond traditional methods of treating dog health issues and presents a comprehensive viewpoint that values the relationship between nature and well-being.

This informative guide carefully selects a wealth of herbal knowledge to address a wide range of canine health issues. These herbs are a gift from Mother Nature to our devoted friends, providing everything from strengthening the immune system to relieving joint pain. Each chapter presents the benefits of each herb in detail, along with instructions on how to incorporate them into your dog's daily routine. Each chapter flows with accuracy.

"Medicinal Herbs for Canine Well-Being" stands out due to its dedication to accessibility and clarity. This book makes sure that integrating medicinal herbs into your dog's routine is a fun and fulfilling experience, regardless of your level of experience with herbal remedies or your level of curiosity about the benefits of natural healing.

The captivating story transports you to the verdant landscapes of herbal medicine, demystifying intricate concepts and giving you hope that you can properly care for your dog. With the help of this invaluable guide, enjoy the transformational force of nature, where the relationship between a guardian and their dog blossoms in the embrace of healing herbs.

This fascinating investigation into the realm of herbal treatments provides the necessary overall quality for your dog's well-being. "Medicinal Herbs for Canine Well-Being" is essential because the interplay between nature and nurture plays a complex role in your dog's health.

HAPPY IMPLEMENTATION

EXECUTION IS RESULT!!

www.ingramcontent.com/pod-product-compliance
Lightning Source LLC
Chambersburg PA
CBHW050849260726
48660CB00006B/2525